First Aid for the Beginner

The Basics of First Aid

I0435658

Prepping and Survival Series

M. Usman

Mendon Cottage Books

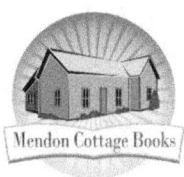

JD-Biz Publishing

All Rights Reserved.

No part of this publication may be reproduced in any form or by any means, including scanning, photocopying, or otherwise without prior written permission from JD-Biz Corp Copyright © 2014

All Images Licensed by Fotolia and 123RF.

Disclaimer

The information is this book is provided for informational purposes only. It is not intended to be used and medical advice or a substitute for proper medical treatment by a qualified health care provider. The information is believed to be accurate as presented based on research by the author.

The contents have not been evaluated by the U.S. Food and Drug Administration or any other Government or Health Organization and the contents in this book are not to be used to treat cure or prevent disease.

The author or publisher is not responsible for the use or safety of any diet, procedure or treatment mentioned in this book. The author or publisher is not responsible for errors or omissions that may exist.

Warning

The Book is for informational purposes only and before taking on any diet, treatment or medical procedure, it is recommended to consult with your primary health care provider.

Our books are available at

1. Amazon.com
2. Barnes and Noble
3. Itunes
4. Kobo
5. Smashwords
6. Google Play Books

Table of Contents

Introduction

When it comes to defining first aid, it means the immediate care provided to an ill or injured person before a proper medical treatment is availed. In other words, first aid can be regarded as the life saving measures. But, why is it so important to know about first aid? The main purpose of first aid is to save the lives of people in life threatening accidental situations when no help is around. No doubt, the era we live in is the era of technologies, machines and modern vehicles, but unfortunately we are utilizing these facilities at the cost of our precious lives. The incidences of fire cases and road side accidents have been increasing for the past few decades. But, in most of the accidental situations, the death of the victim happens due to the lack of immediate medical treatment. Sometimes, it is not possible for the ambulance or a doctor to reach to the calamity stricken location immediately. What would you do if a friend of yours was choking in front of you and none of the people are around you was a doctor? Obviously, you just wouldn't let your friend die in front of your eyes. This is where your training or knowledge of first aid would come handy, if you had any. By knowing the first aid skills, you might be at least able to save the life of victims on the spot before help could arrive. This clearly portrays the importance of first aid training. The number of precious lives that we lose every year in accidents can be significantly reduced by promoting the concept of first aid training.

This basic purpose of this book is to teach you different techniques and maneuvers that everyone should at least have some knowledge about. Who knows when you might face an emergency? It's better to be prepared than not. So, buckle your seat belts and dive into the world of handy first aid skills that you should know. I'm sure by the time you reach the end of this book, you'll be happy that you came across something this good.

Chapter 1 – Getting Started

You happen to be present in a calamity stricken spot. People are lucky to have you around since you have some know how about first aid. But, before jumping into the situation to be a hero, you should keep some important things in mind.

Objectives of first aid

Before you can even start with first aid you should know what objectives first aid serves. These objectives include:

- To rescue victim's life.

- To protect him and to preclude further injury from occurring.

- To help the victim in recovery or healing.

Keep in mind!

- Call the concerned authorities (like 911) without wasting a single second. The more you delay your call for help, the more deleterious would be the outcome. Tell the emergency support center about all essentials like the incident, the place of incident, and severity of situation.

- After assessing the whole situation, carefully observe the victim. Note the vital signs like breathing, pulse, and temperature.

- Check the consciousness of the victim. You can give voice commands to the victim for assessing whether he is unconscious, drowsy, or alert.

- It's only when the victim is unconscious or not responding that you go for airway ventilation, breathing management, and cardiopulmonary resuscitation.

Personal safety comes first!

You might be waiting desperately to save lives of the victims, but remember that personal safety comes first. You should keep in mind following points:

- Use Nitrile gloves (if you have some) before handling the victim.

- At least cover the mouth of the victim with a cloth before doing mouth to mouth breathing.

- Be careful while using sharp objects and tools.

- Avoid getting in direct contact with body fluids and blood of the victim.

- Carefully assess the surrounding area for dangers like electricity wires or falling bricks. No one would come to rescue you if you were reckless enough to jump into a difficult situation. If you feel that giving first aid would put your life in danger, don't go near the victim and wait for authorities to come.

Chapter 2 – First Aid for Airway Obstruction

Most of the time, the victims you come across will be in an unconscious state. The major problem faced in unconscious victims is airway obstruction or breathing difficulty. In a normal or conscious person, the muscles that control the movement of the tongue are in a tensed state. This prevents the tongue from falling back or closing the respiratory inlet in the throat. But, the opposite happens in an unconscious person and that leads to airway obstruction. When the person is unconscious, the tongue muscles are relaxed and the tongue tends to fall back. It is the falling back of the tongue that is responsible for obstructing the airway. The unconscious person is also more prone to inhale the vomitus or coming from the stomach, which may further aggravate the airway obstruction. Maintaining a patent airway is the first challenge that is faced while resuscitating the unconscious casualty. Sometimes, the unconscious victim dies on the spot, not due to the primary injuries, but due to the secondary airway obstruction. If the airway obstruction persists for 5-6 min, the patient may die due to lack of oxygen supply to the brain. That's why the first thing you need to do while saving the unconscious person is to look for the airway obstruction, before paying attention to other injuries.

Several methods to manage the airway obstruction are:

Finger sweep method

The finger sweep method is done on unconscious victims to clear the air passage of any foreign body or food debris that you can actually see.

- Make the victim lie down on a flat surface in a face up (supine) position.

- Once the victim is in position, try to open the mouth of the victim by grasping his lower jaw and tongue between thumb and finger. While grasping the lower jaw, slightly lift it. This tongue-jaw lifting action will draw the tongue away from the back of the throat, making it easier for you to look inside and to locate the foreign body.

- After locating the foreign body, insert your index finger into the victim's mouth and slide it carefully along the side of cheek towards the base of the tongue.

- Now make a hook of finger and gently sweep across the throat to remove the foreign body. You need to be careful while sweeping the finger; otherwise the foreign body can be driven deep into the airway.

Head tilt/ chin lift method

The other method for maintaining the airway patent is head tilt/chin lift maneuver. This maneuver is especially important when you can't see the thing obstructing the airways.

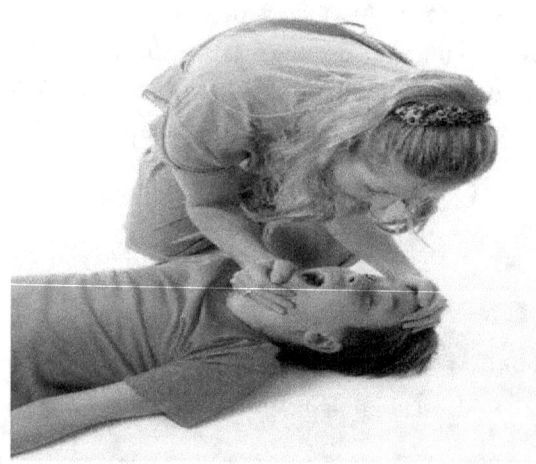

Kneel on one side of victim (preferably on the right side). The victim must be lying in a face up position. Place your one hand firmly on the forehead of the victim. Now gently apply backward pressure on the forehead. As a result of this action, the neck will be extended. But, be careful and do not apply too much pressure on the head as extending the neck beyond its limit may lead to spinal injuries or fractures. Also, keep in mind that this maneuver should not be done on victims with suspected head or neck injury (all victims of a fall or road side accident should be dealt with as spinal injury case). While keeping one hand on the forehead, place the thumb and index finger of the other hand on the bony prominence of the chin. Never apply pressure on the soft tissues of chin because it can further obstruct the airway. Now lift the chin up and hold it in this position. Avoid closing the mouth as it can prevent the air from entering into the mouth. This head tilt/ chin lift method helps in keeping the airway open by pulling the tongue away from the back of the throat.

Jaw thrust method

Jaw thrust method is preferred in victims having suspected head and neck injuries or fractures, because there is no need of extending or moving the neck in this maneuver. First kneel near the head of the victim. Then, with the help of fingers (not thumbs) of both hands, grasp the angle of the lower jaw and lift it up. Continue lifting the jaw until the lower jaw and teeth are displaced forward to the upper jaw teeth. After that, with the help of your free thumbs depress this elevated jaw. This should open the airway.

Chapter 3 – First Aid for Breathing

How to assess breathing trouble?

The first step is to assess whether the victim you've come across is breathing or not. You can do the following steps to check the breathing difficulty in the victim:

- Carefully, look for the chest movements. No visible chest movements indicate there isn't any breathing or difficulty in breathing.

- Bring your face or cheek near the victim's nostrils and feel the breath of the victim.

- Place your ear on the chest of the victim and listen to the breathing sounds. Absence of breathing sounds or abnormal sounds indicate breathing difficulty.

How to maintain the breathing?

If you see that the victim is having difficulty breathing, waste no time in starting the emergency maneuver for maintaining the breathing. Here are some simple and quick methods to rescue the breathing:

Mouth to mouth breathing

This is the most basic thing that you can try to rescue a person with little or no breathing. This technique might sound gross to you, but trust me this simple maneuver can help you save precious lives. Mouth to mouth breathing consists of following basic steps:

- Make the victim lie flat on his back (supine position). Kneel on one side of the victim (preferably to the right). If the victim is wearing any tight clothing or collar, loosen it quickly.

- Open the mouth of the victim and clear the throat by sweeping through a finger.

- Perform head tilt/chin lift maneuver.

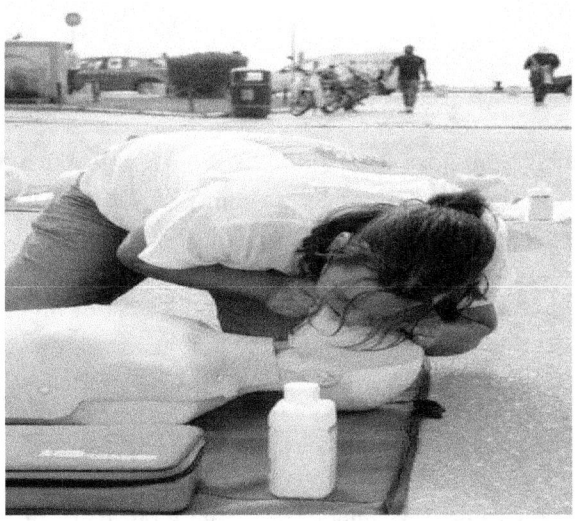

- Close the nostrils of the victim with the help of your index finger and thumb of the hand that is resting or applying pressure on the forehead. This stops the leaking of air through nostrils during the maneuver.

- Cover the mouth of the victim with a piece of cloth and take a deep breath to inhale as much air as possible.

- After inhaling the air, place your mouth on the victim's mouth. Your lips must be sealed with victim's lips to prevent the escape of air.

- Blow air hard into the victim's mouth. Give 10 breaths per minute at the rate of 1 breath per 5 or 6 second.

- Simultaneously, look at the victim's chest for breathing movements. Continue doing this until the chest rises. If the chest movement occurs, remove your mouth and let the victim breathe. Bring your face near the victim's nostrils and feel his breath.

Mouth to nose breathing

Mouth to mouth breathing method cannot be performed on victims having jaw fractures, lip injuries and jaw spasms. Under these circumstances, mouth to nose breathing is preferred.

- Place the victim in supine posture and perform head tilt/chin lift maneuver.

- Cover the victim nose with a piece of cloth. Now take a deep breath and place your mouth around the victim's nose. Your mouth must be sealed around the nose of the victim.

- Now blow the air forcefully into his nose. Keep his mouth slightly open to let the air escape through the mouth.

- Continue doing this until the victim resumes his breathing. 10 breathes per minute should be given.

- After giving 10 breaths, check the victim's pulse and heartbeat. If the pulse is still low, continue the artificial breathing or perform the CPR (cardiopulmonary resuscitation)

Mouth to mouth breathing for infants and children

- Position the child in a supine position and perform head tilt/ chin lift maneuver. But, avoid applying too much pressure on child's head as it can further obstruct the airway.

- Cover the child's mouth with a piece of cloth and seal your mouth around the child's mouth. Now blow the air into the child's mouth. The blowing of air should not be as hard as done while resuscitating an adult person. The lungs of children and infants are delicate, so over inflating the lungs can cause injury to them.

- If the chest of the child rises, stop blowing the air and let the chest fall. Give one breath per three seconds until the victim starts breathing.

- Keep checking the pulse of the child. If the pulse is lower than normal continue doing the procedure. If the pulse still remains low, go for CPR.

Chapter 4 – First Aid for Choking

The windpipe is the only way through which the air can enter into the lungs. The obstruction of this wind pipe, at any level, may lead to choking. Choking occurs when a either a foreign body or food gets lodged into the windpipe. The obstruction of the windpipe prevents the air from reaching the lungs, leading to the lack of oxygen in the body. Since lungs are the only way for oxygen to enter into the body, the persistence of choking for a few minutes can deplete your body of oxygen. The vital organs of the body, like the brain and heart, need a continuous supply of oxygen to function properly. But, the brain responds more sensitively to the low oxygen level in the body and responds as unconsciousness or irreversible damage to the brain cells.

Choking is a commonly faced medical emergency. It can either be complete or partial depending upon the extent of blockage. The victim of choking can be recognized by following signs:

- Inability to speak

- Difficulty in breathing

- Gasping and wheezing

- Hands clutching the throat

- Bluish discoloration of skin, lips and nails (signs of cyanosis)

- Altered consciousness

The first aid intervention of choking depends upon the degree of choking, consciousness and responsiveness of the victim. The first aid strategies are different for both partial and complete obstruction.

Ask the victim to cough

First, check if the victim is conscious or not. If the victim is conscious then give him some voice commands. If the person responds, it means there is only partial obstruction of the airway. In such cases, there is no need to go for complex maneuvers like abdominal thrusts and chest thrusts. You can simply ask the patient to cough out the body causing obstruction. Doing any other method can push the foreign body further down the airway, causing more obstruction.

Back blows

If the victim is unable to expel out the foreign body with coughing, give him five back blows immediately. First stand behind the choking person. Ask him to lean forward. Then, with the heel of your hand, give 5 back blows between the two blades of the shoulder. Never forget to ask the victim to lean forward as it aids the dislodged foreign body to come out through the mouth rather than going down the airway.

Abdominal thrust (Heimlich maneuver)

Complete obstruction or choking is an emergency condition that needs to be relieved immediately, otherwise the victim can expire.

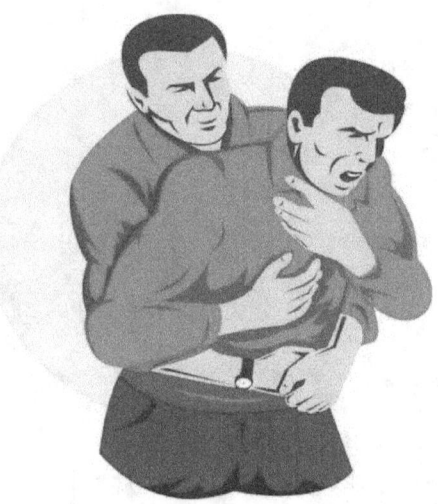

If you see that the victim is conscious, first try giving back blows. But if it fails to relieve the obstruction, go for the Heimlich maneuver or abdominal thrusts.

<u>When the patient is standing</u>

- Stand behind the victim. Wrap your arms around the victim's abdomen.

- Make the victim lean forward as it will prevent the foreign body from being pushed further down the airway.

- Now make a fist of your one hand and place it at the midpoint between the tip of the sternum (breast bone) and umbilicus. Using your other hand, grasp your fist firmly.

- Give sharp thrusts in the upward and inward direction like you are trying to lift him up. When the thrust is applied, the pressure on the diaphragm increases, which in turn compresses the lung. The air present within the compressed lungs tries to be expelled out by force or pressure. This pressurized air then assists in pushing the foreign body out through the mouth.

- Meantime keep looking into the mouth for any visible obstruction. If you can locate the foreign object coming out through the throat, use the finger sweep technique to take it out of the victim's throat.

When the patient is lying

- The victim must be lying in a supine position. Then straddle the victim's legs.

- Lean forward over the victim. Place the heel of one hand in the midline between the umbilicus and the xiphoid process (tip of the breast bone).

- Keep your hand in a fixed position by supporting it with the help of your other hand.

- While keeping your elbows straight, apply pressure or thrust in the upward and inward direction.

- Repeat the thrusts 5-6 times until the foreign body dislodges or comes out of the airway.

- If the victim vomits out the obstructing object, turn the victim's head to one side and do the finger sweep to clear the throat.

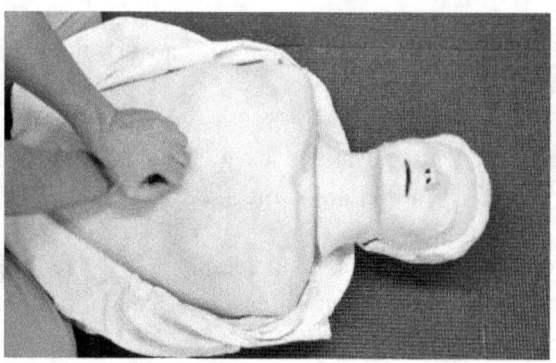

Chest thrusts

Heimlich maneuver or abdominal thrusts are not recommended for obese victims and pregnant women. In such victims, chest thrusts are advised. The proper way to do chest thrusts is as follows:

- Make the victim to lie in the supine position. Place yourself on the one side of the victim.

- Place the heel of one hand on the base of breastbone of the victim. Now place your other hand on the top of the first hand to support it.

- By keeping your arms straight, give thrusts in the upward and inward direction. Repeat the method till the obstructing object comes out.

Choking management in infants and children

The airway in children is more prone to obstruction because it is more straight and short as compared to the airway in adults. If you come across a choking emergency in children or infants, the back slaps and chest thrusts must be performed immediately to relieve it. First of all, you should sit down somewhere. Now place the child in a face downward position on your thigh. The head should be slightly lower than the level of the shoulders as it will help the obstructing material to come out easily. Support the head of the child with one hand and give five gentle back slaps or blows between the shoulder blades with the help of other hand. After that, look into the mouth of the child to clear away foreign materials.

If the choking is not relieved on giving five back slaps, go for the chest thrusts. The chest thrusts can be given with the same technique as given in the adults. But, the position of the child is important while giving chest thrusts. The child should be placed in the lap with the head lower than the trunk. Then place two fingers at the base of the sternum or breastbone, fixing them firmly by placing the palm of the other hand on them. Give 5 sharp thrusts until the obstruction is relieved.

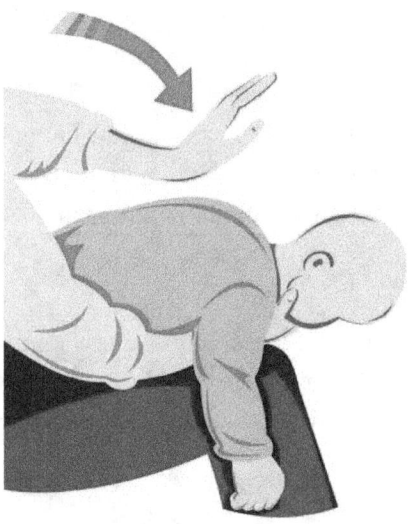

If the child's age is above than one year, the abdominal thrusts can be done. But the abdominal thrusts are not recommended for infants, as the infant's abdominal organs are more prone to get injured during abdominal thrusts.

Chapter 5 – Cardiopulmonary Resuscitation (CPR)

Cardiopulmonary resuscitation is the maneuver done in emergency situations when the victim is unconscious, not responding, or not breathing due to cardiac arrest. Cardiac arrest is a very serious condition in which the heart stops working. The heart keeps pumping the blood to every part of the body throughout the whole life of a person. But, when the heart stops working the blood flow to the vital organs stops. If the heart remains in arrest for more than 4 minutes, the victim can die. Cardiac arrest can happen due to many reasons like atrial and ventricular fibrillations, shock, asphyxia and heart attack. The purpose of doing cardiopulmonary resuscitation is to maintain the blood flow and the breathing in the victimized person.

How to do CPR?

There are two components of CPR technique: chest compressions for forcing the heart to pump and mouth to mouth rescue breaths for maintaining the respiration and oxygenation in the body tissues.

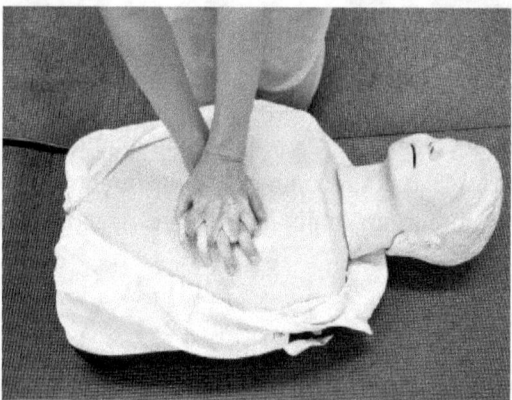

The steps of CPR are as follows:

- Kneel beside the victim, close to his chest.

- Locate the point where you have to apply the compressions. Run two fingers of one hand along the lower border of ribs. Find out the point where the ribs meet the breastbone.

- Now place the heel of one hand on the point of compression. This point lies approximately at the base or lower part of the breastbone or sternum.

- Place your other hand on the top of the first hand (left hand would lie on top on the right hand if you're a right handed). Interlock the fingers with each other, but keep them off the chest wall. Only the heels of the hands should be resting on the compression point.

- Now push the chest down with pressure. The chest should go in up to 2 inches in each compression. While giving the compression, the arms should be kept straight, elbows locked and your whole body weight should be supported on the arms and hands. After each compression, release the pressure on the sternum without taking your hand off the chest wall. Let the chest wall recoil and relax. But, the time intervals of both compression and relaxation should be the same.

- The chest compression rate should be 100 compressions per 1 minute. After every 30 compressions, give two rescue breaths. Make the airway patent by tilting the head and lifting the chin. Pinch the nose of the victim and give two mouth to mouth breaths (same maneuvers as mentioned before).

- After every two minutes, assess the victim's situation by palpating his carotid pulse. If the victim is still not responding or breathing, continue doing the CPR until the medical facility is availed.

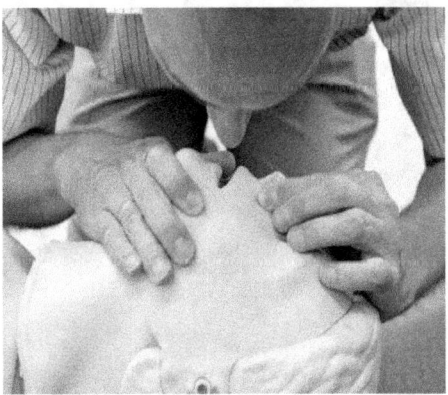

CPR in children

For children above the age of one year

- Place the heel of one hand in the middle of the chest at the junction of the sternum and ribs.

- Push the chest down by 3 cm or 1 inch. It should not be more than this because the child's ribs are more prone to fracture during CPR.

- Maintain the compression rate of 100 compressions per minute. After 30 compresses, give two mouth to mouth breaths.

- After two minutes of compressions, check the child's carotid pulse and feel the breath. If the condition does not improve, continue doing the CPR.

For children below the age of one year (infants)

The other steps are the same as done in adults and children above the age of 1 year. But, in infants the two finger method is preferred because the ribs of infants are delicate and are unable to bear excessive pressure. Place the index finger and middle finger of one hand in the middle of the chest just below the nipple line of the child. Now compress the chest by 2 cm by applying pressure through two fingers. After 30 compresses, give two rescue breaths. Keep doing it till the child revives.

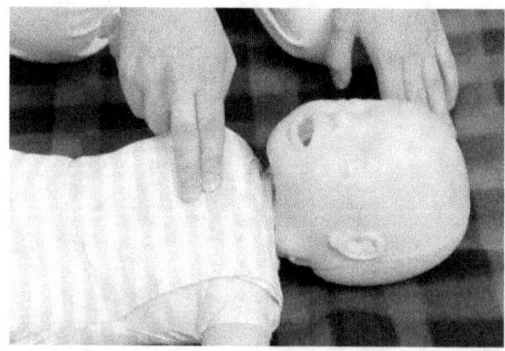

Chapter 6 – First Aid for Bleeding

Bleeding complications are commonly faced in road side accidents and even at home. Loss of too much blood (more than 1 liter) can lead to low blood volume and ultimately the death of the victim. Following measures can be taken to avoid massive blood loss:

Direct pressure

- Carefully observe the site of wound or bleeding. If there is any foreign object sticking into the wound, carefully separate ut. But never try to scratch the cloth that sticks to the wound because it can cause more injury to the bleeding wound.

- Take a sterile bandage and wrap it around the wound firmly. Continue applying direct pressure on the wound until the bleeding stops.

- If the dressing soaks all the blood, do not try to remove. Instead, wrap more dressings or gauzes around it to maintain the pressure.

- Continue applying pressure on the wound. It is advised to wear gloves before you stop bleeding because you can get an infection from the wound of the victim. Do wash hand afterwards.

- If the bleeding occurs from wounds in the arms and legs, elevate the affected part above the level of the heart. This will help in reducing the oozing of blood from the wound.

Compress the pressure points

If the bleeding does not stop on applying direct pressure, the other way to stop the bleeding is compressing the main artery supplying that area. Some important pressure points in the body are:

- For bleeding in the arm the pressure point is the upper part of the arm beneath the armpit.

- For the forearm the pressure point is on the inner side of the arm just above the elbow.

- For the hand, the wrist is the pressure point.

- The groin region and back of the knee are the pressure points for leg bleeding.

- For the bleeding of the skull, the pressure point is on the temple and for the face, bleeding below the level of the eyes pressure can be applied at the base of the jaw bone.

- For controlling the bleeding of the neck, compress the carotid vessel located slightly away from the mid line of the neck

Tourniquet

Tourniquets are stretchable, constricting bands that are tied tightly just above the wound to prevent the bleeding. But the tourniquet should be used only when there is a risk to the victim's life.

Chapter 7 – First Aid for Poisoning

Poisoning can be accidental, suicidal and homicidal. Poisoned victims may show signs of drowsiness, confusion, difficulty in breathing, foul smelling breath, bruises or wounds around the lips and mouth, bluish coloration of the face, convulsions, cool clammy skin and a feeble pulse. But, the appearance of symptoms varies with the type of poison and the route of entry of the poison in the body. The poison can be inhaled, ingested or absorbed through skin. Therefore, the first aid management of poisoning also varies accordingly:

For ingested poison

- First, assess the victim. Look for burns and wounds around the mouth and lips.

- Check the victim's mouth. If there is any vomitus, turn his head to one side and do the finger sweep to take out the vomitus.

- Do not try to induce vomiting, especially in unconscious victims. If the clothes are contaminated with poison, remove them and wash the skin with water.

- If the person is unconscious and not breathing, start CPR immediately.

- Keep the person warm and comfortable. Immediately shift the casualty to the nearby hospital or poison center for proper management.

For inhaled poison

- Move the person away from the poisonous or suffocating environment. Get him into the fresh air as soon as possible.

- While doing so, protect yourself from inhaling the poisonous fumes. Wrap a cloth around your mouth and nose.

- After rescuing the person, maintain his airway, breathing and pulse. If the person is not responding, go for CPR immediately.

For poison in the eyes

- If poison enters the eyes, wash the eyes with cold water for 15-20 minutes and then seek medical help.

For poison on the skin

- Remove the poisoned clothing first.

- Then wash the affected area with water and soap. Do this for 15-20 minutes.

- Avoid getting in contact with the poison.

Chapter 8 – First Aid for Burns

Depending upon the degree of severity, the burns are divided into the following categories:

1st degree burns

These burns affect only the superficial layer of skin, causing redness and mild pain. Place the burned area under running water for 10 minutes. Then apply an antibiotic cream like silver sulfadiazine on the affected area and wrap it with a sterile dressing.

2nd degree burns

Second degree burns penetrate through all the layers of the skin. The symptoms of second degree burns are extreme pain, blister formation and redness of skin. To take care of the second degree burns, follow the given steps:

- Removing the clothing or jewelry, if any, from the burned area.

- Now keep the affected area under running tap water for 10-15 minutes. The cooling effect of water will stop the burn from spreading into the deeper layers of skin.

- Let the burned area dry. Once the burn is dry, apply an antibiotic cream and then gently cover it with a dry and sterile dressing.

- If the burns are on the arms and legs, slightly elevating them can reduce the swelling and edema.

3rd degree burns

Third degree burns are the most severe ones, as they penetrate through the skin layer and damage the underlying tissues like bone, muscles, and nerves. If the person loses too much fluid and blood, he may die of dehydration. Do not remove the clothing of the victim. The burned area should not be kept under cold water. Just cover the affected area very carefully and gently with a sterile dressing. Move to the nearby hospital immediately.

Chapter 9 – First Aid for Fractures and Dislocation

There are many different types of fractures and dislocations. Most of them can be stabilized right after they happen, before medical attention can be sought. Here are a few steps to help stabilize:

- First look for any wound, injury or bleeding. If there is bleeding, stop it by wrapping the wound with a dressing.

- Immobilize the affected part as soon as possible because moving it can aggravate the fracture or dislocation.

- Apply ice packs on the affected area for 10-15 minutes. This helps in reducing the pain and inflammation associated with fracture.

- Now the next step is to stabilize the broken bone. There is no need to fix or realign the broken bone as it requires professional expertise.

- The fractured bone can be stabilized with the help of splints and slings.

- Anything like cardboard, tree sticks and newspapers can be used as a splint. Apply one splint above the fractured bone and one below it. Now keep these splints fixed by tying them with a tie or a piece of cloth.

- Put a padding of cloth or towel between the splints to avoid pressure on the fractured bone.

  - If the fractures are of the arm and forearm, the best thing you can do to completely immobilize the fractured bone is to hang the splinted part with the help of a sling around the neck or shoulder of the other side.

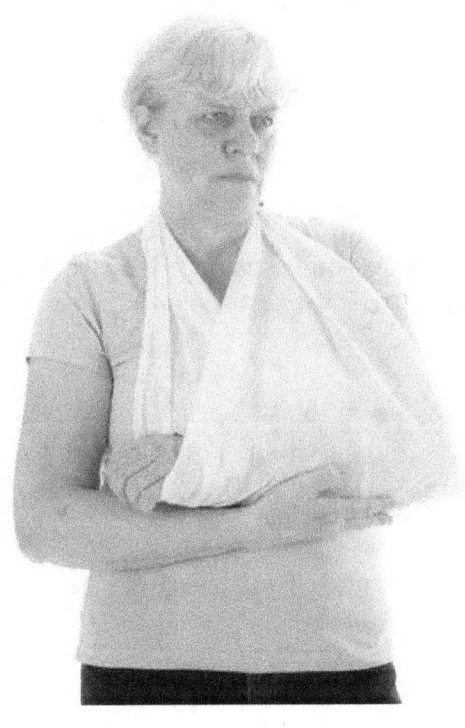

Chapter 10 – First Aid for Shock

Shock is an emergency condition, in which the blood supply to body tissues is significantly reduced. There can be several reasons of shock, like cardiac arrest, blood loss, burns, trauma, spinal injuries and anaphylactic reactions. The signs of shock are: cold clammy skin, pale face, excessive sweating, difficulty in breathing or shallow breathing, nausea, vomiting, feeble pulse and altered conscious.

- Elevate the victim's legs off the ground. This helps in pushing the blood from the peripheral parts of the body to the vital organs like the brain and heart.

- Then, maintain the airway, breathing, and pulse of the victim. If the person is not conscious, do CPR to keep the heart working.

- Wrap the person in a blanket and keep him calm and warm.

- If the person starts vomiting, turn him to one side so the vomitus comes of mouth easily.

- If bleeding is the underlying cause, make efforts to stop it instantly.

- Bring the victim to the hospital for further management.

Chapter 11 – First Aid for Seizures

Seizures can happen at any time, usually with no warning. There are many reasons that people have seizures, most commonly due to medical illnesses. It is a scary situation for everyone involved, but there are a few steps below to try and make it easier to help someone out.

- Make the person lie on a flat surface. Loosen the tight clothing around his neck.

- To protect the person from any injury, remove the nearby furniture and objects or place him away from such objects.

- Try to protect the victim's head.

- If he vomits, turn the head to one side and clear out the vomit with finger.

- Keep the person warm and comfortable until he becomes normal.

Chapter 12 – First Aid for Stings and Bites

Stings of non-poisonous insects may not be deadly, but the bite of creatures like a snake can lead to death. The following steps should be taken to manage stings and bites of insects:

- Keep the person calm and comfortable.

- Monitor the vital signs like pulse, breathing, and heartbeat.

- Immobilize the affected part to prevent the spread of sting poison to other sites.

- Wash the affected part with water and soap. If it is a case of snakebite, take the person immediately to the hospital.

- For the stings of minor insects, the antihistamines can be taken to reduce swelling, allergy, and pain.

Conclusion

First aid is knowledge that every person should have. If more people would learn the basics of first aid, we could possibly save more lives. In this book we have discussed most of the basics of first aid. We have included many areas, and hopefully helped to boost your morale in case you are ever in a situation of being the first responder. Read this book again and again until the basics of first aid are second nature to you. Be sure to share your knowledge with others. Thank you for reading and remember to be safe!

Author Bio

Muhammad Usman is a distinguished medical graduate of Allama Iqbal medical college (AIMC). He is a professional writer who has been in the field for more than 4 years. During this time he has produced 10,000+ articles, blogs and eBooks on various niches related to diseases, health, fitness, nutrition and well-being. He is a regular contributor to several journals related to medicine and surgery. He is the editor of several journals and newspapers.

Check out some of the other JD-Biz Publishing books

Gardening Series on Amazon

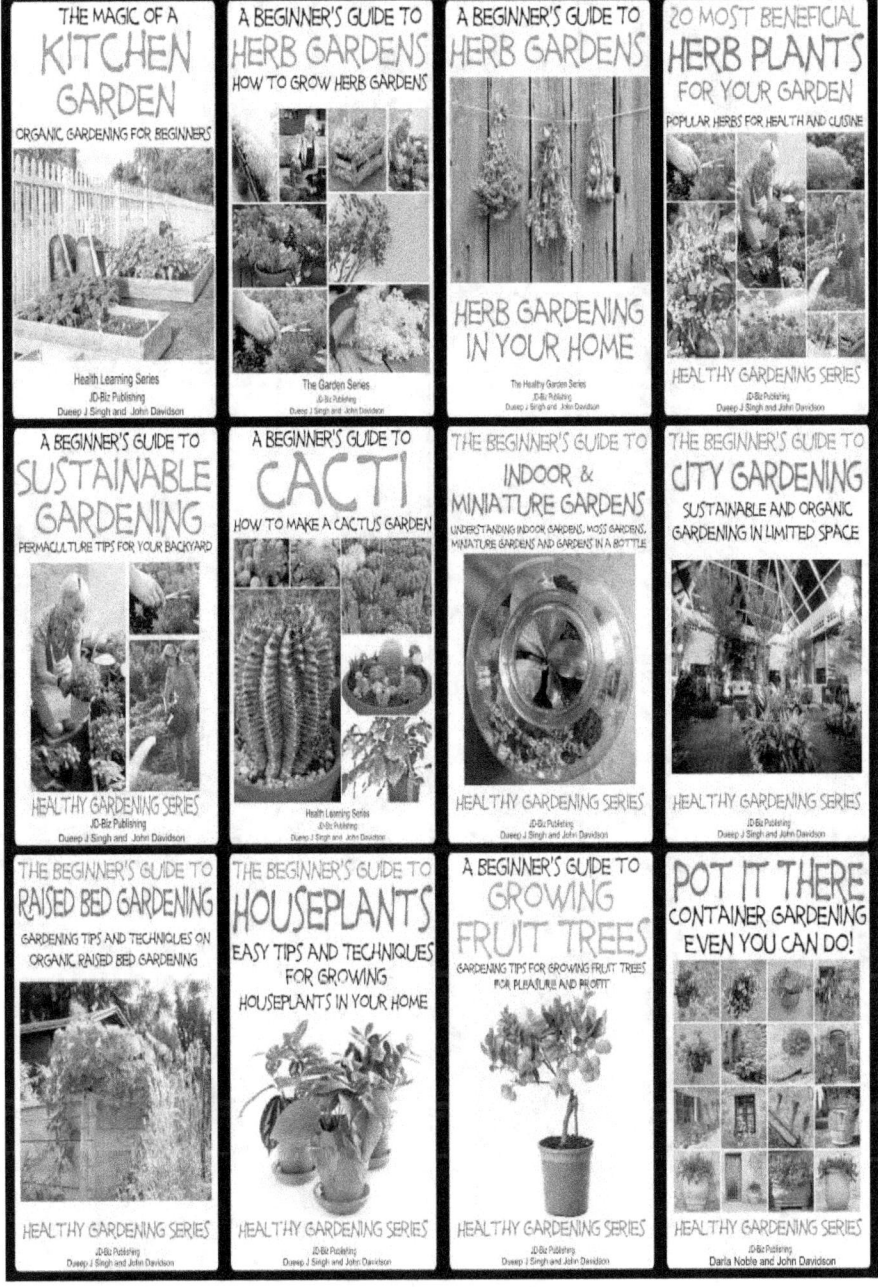

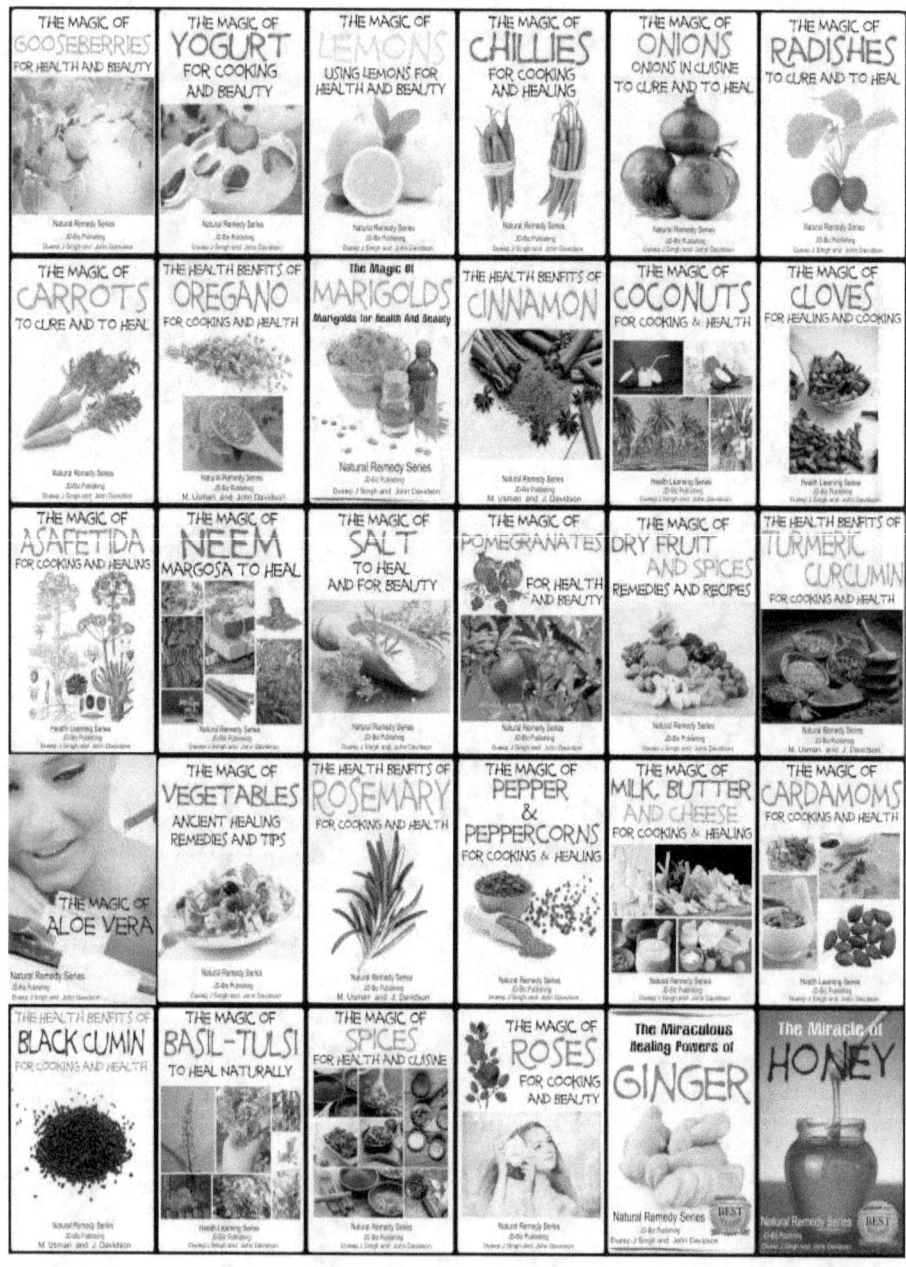

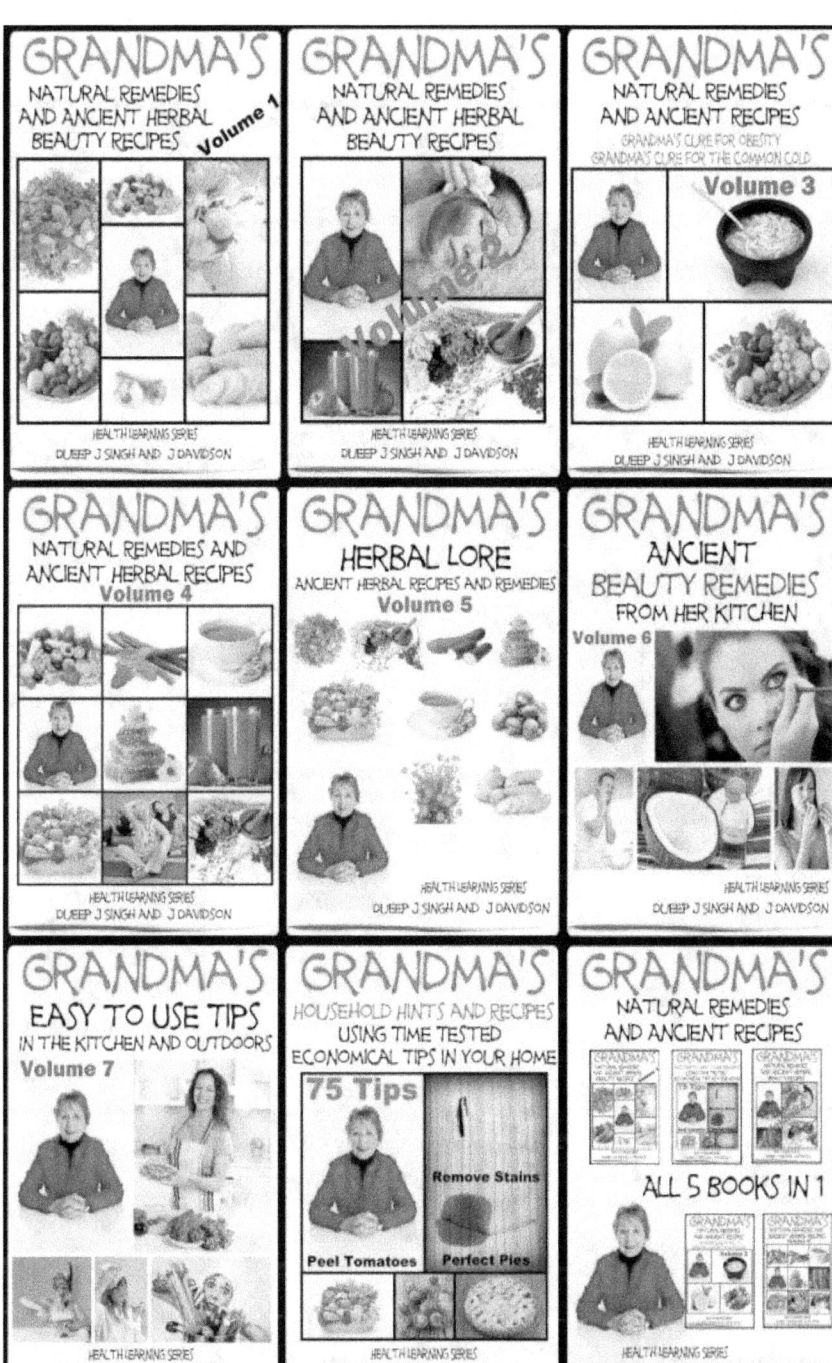

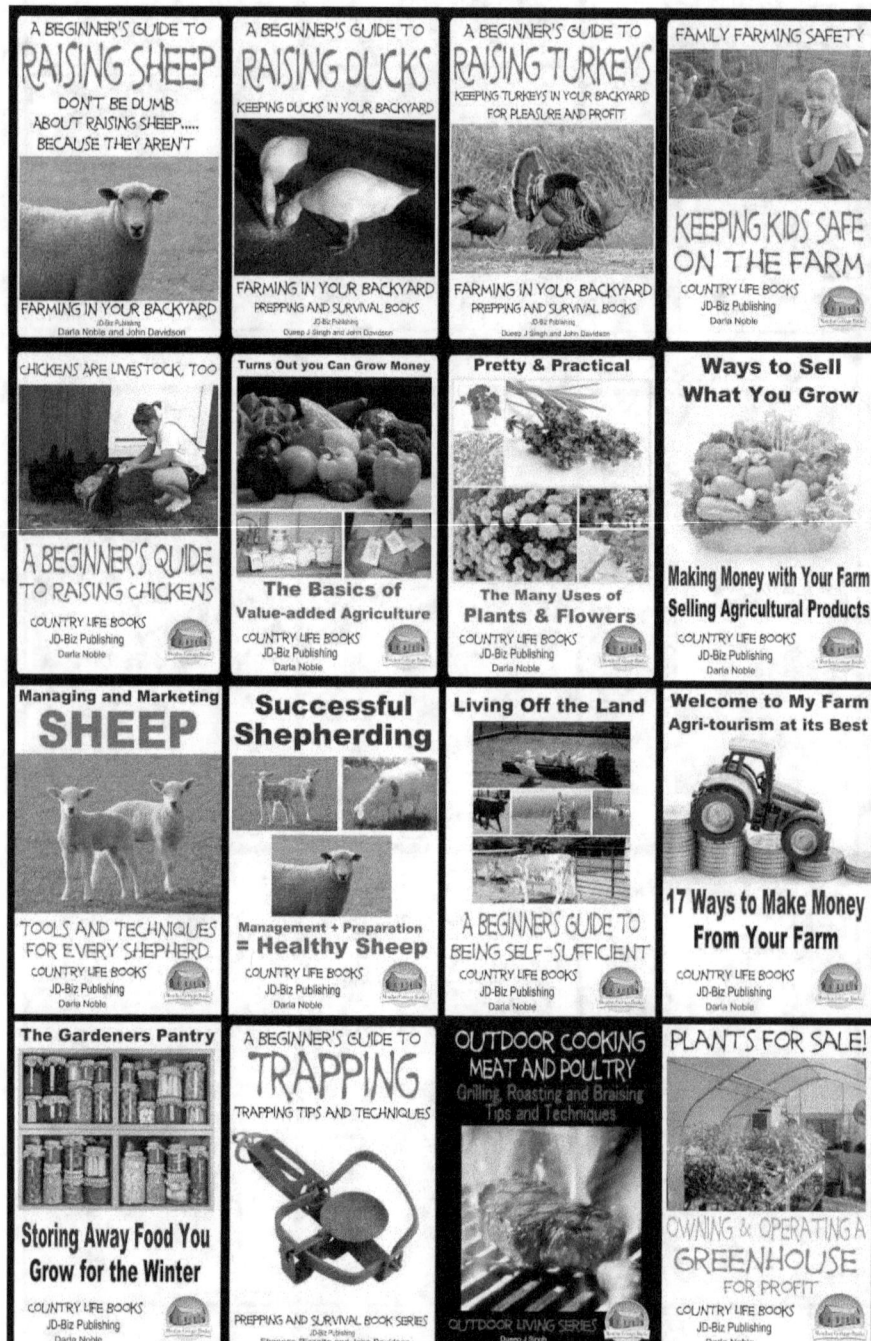

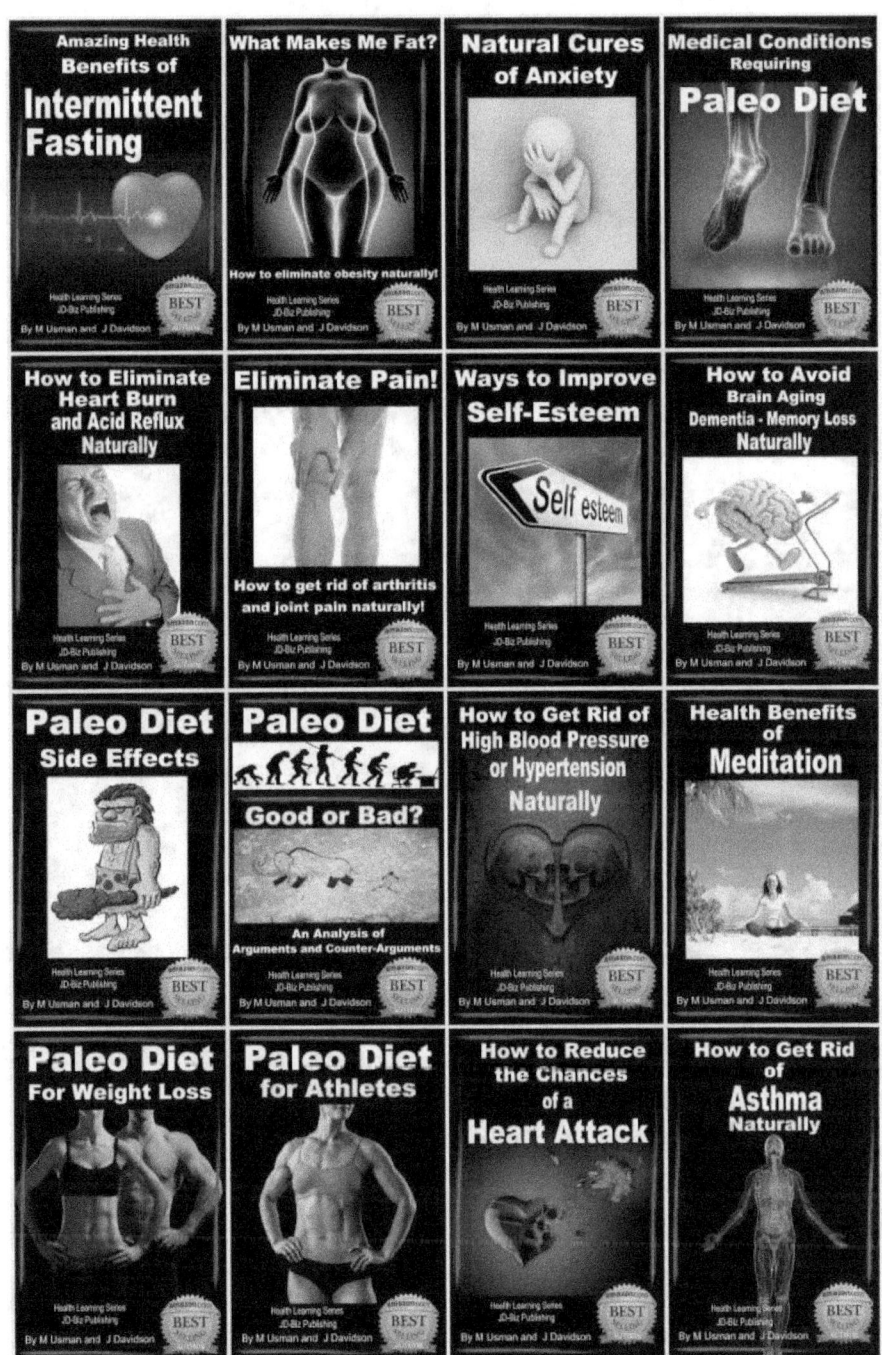

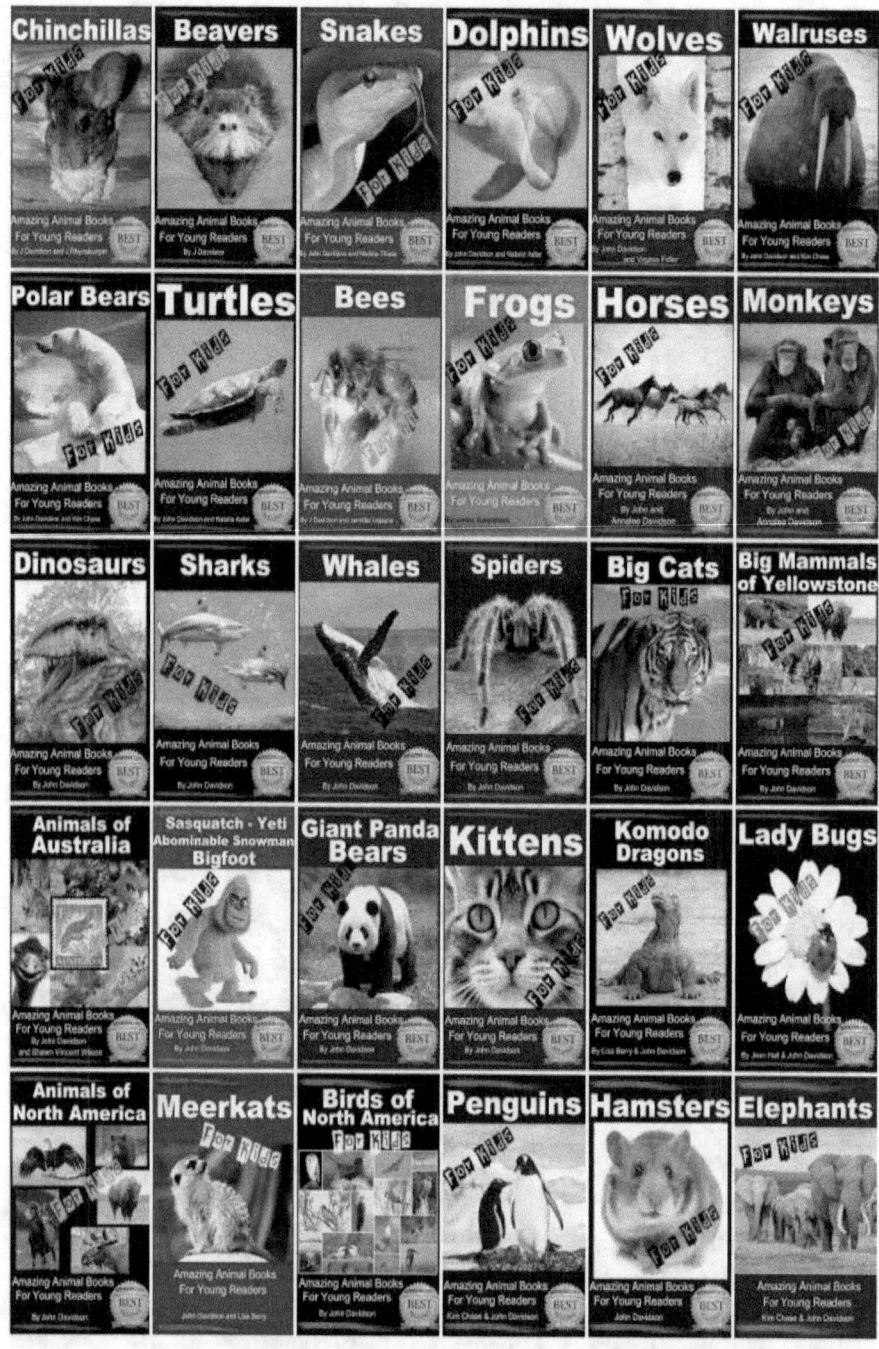

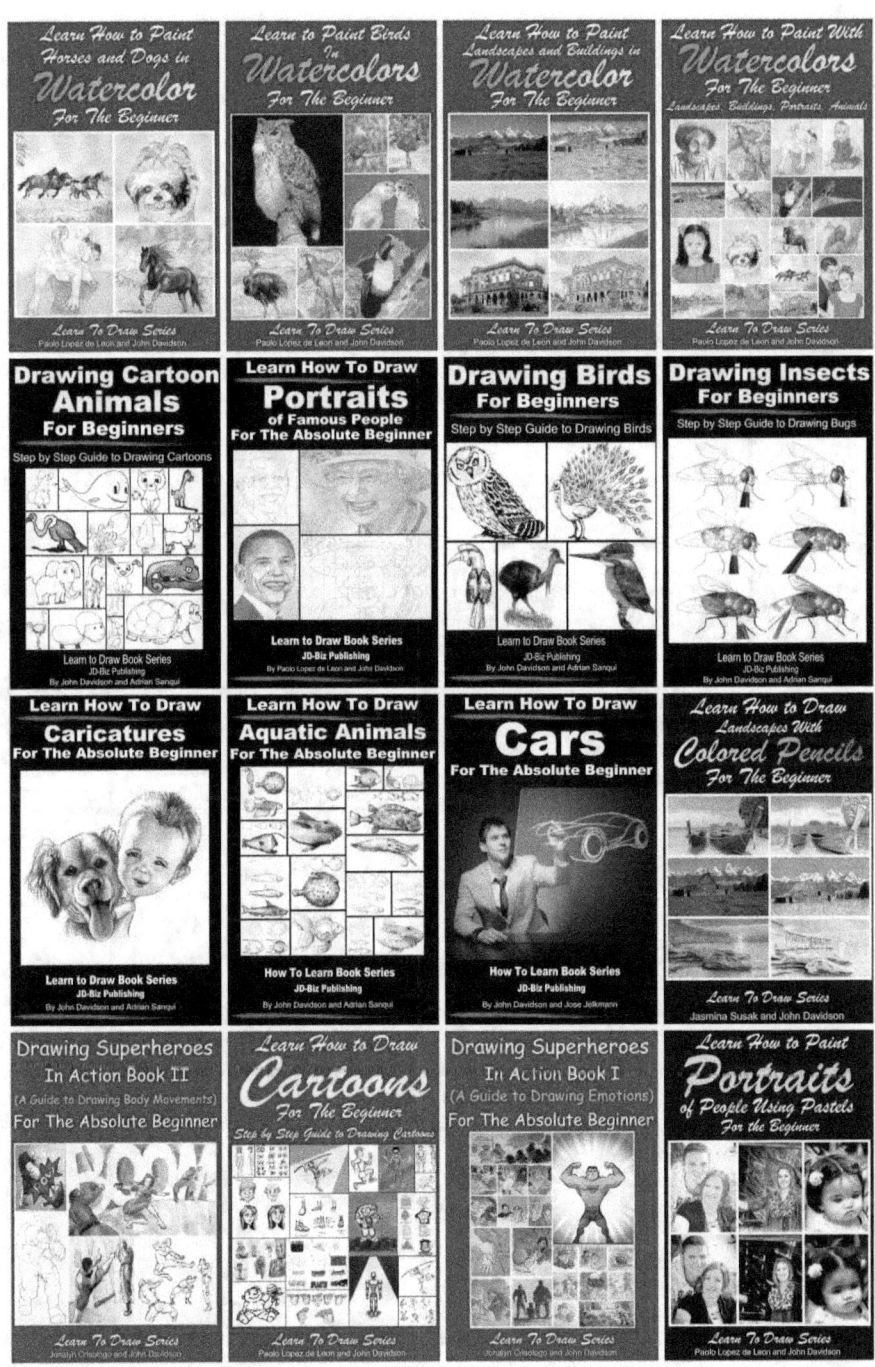

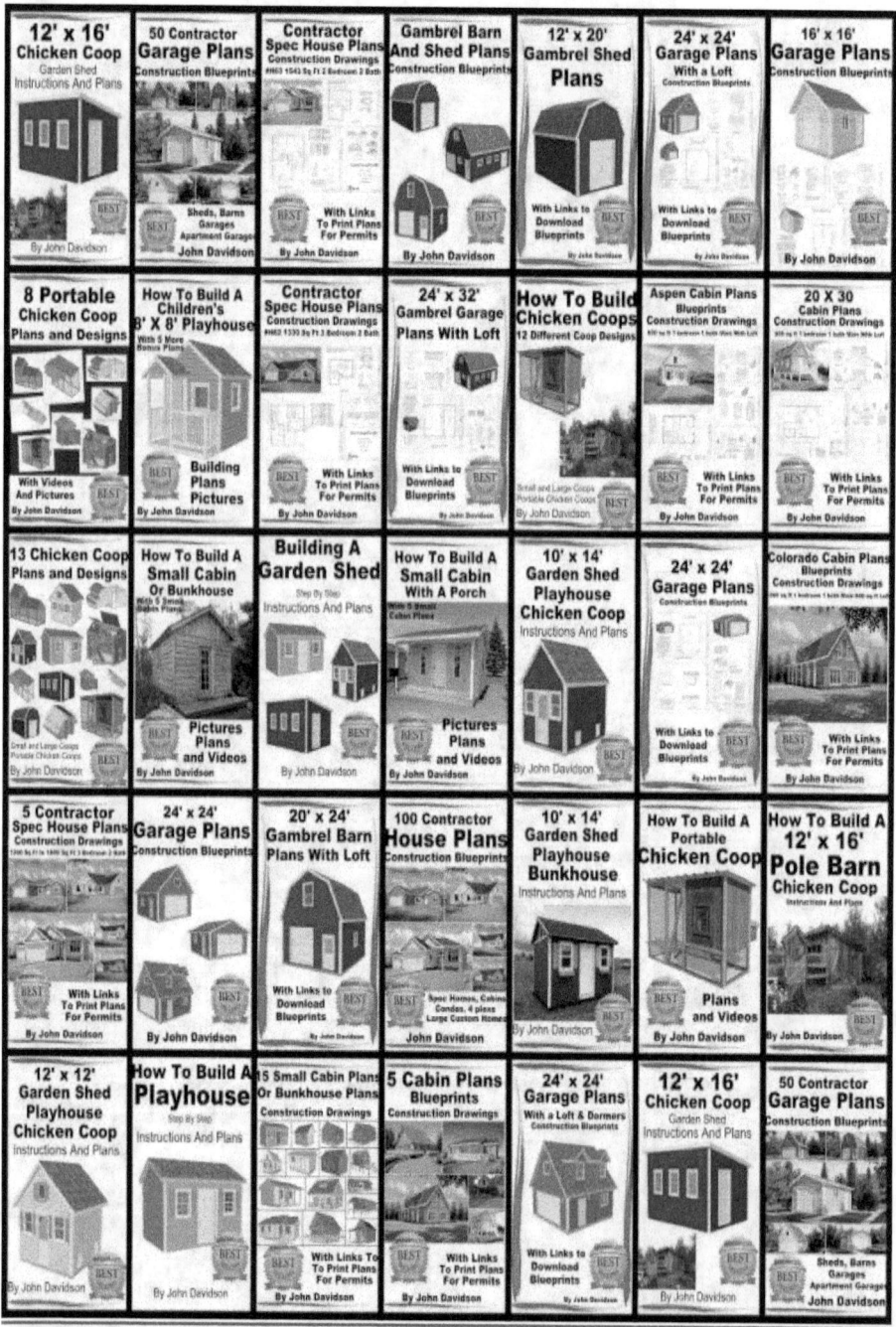

Entrepreneur Book Series

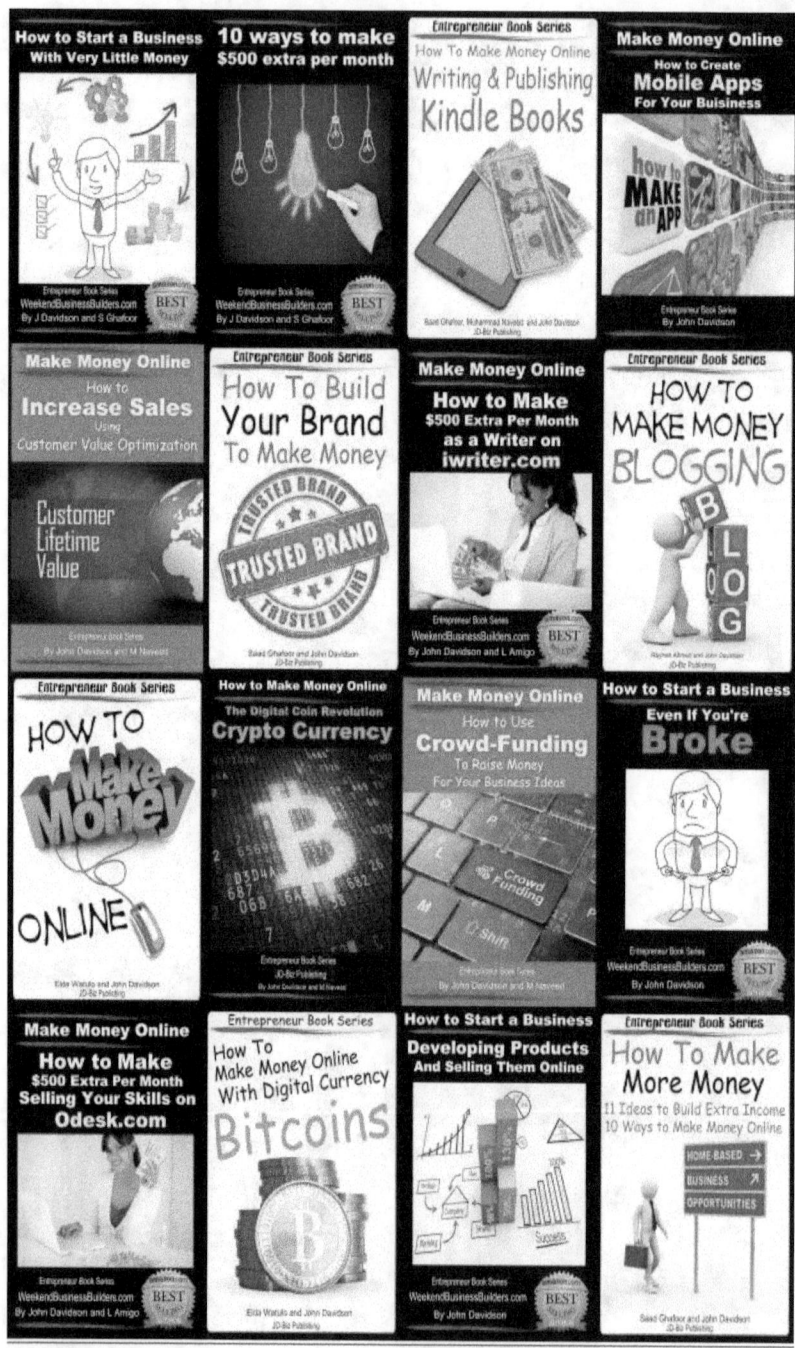

Our books are available at

1. Amazon.com

2. Barnes and Noble

3. Itunes

4. Kobo

5. Smashwords

6. Google Play Books

Publisher

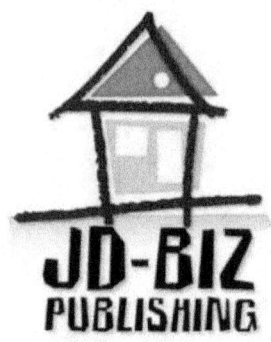

JD-Biz Corp

P O Box 374

Mendon, Utah 84325

http://www.jd-biz.com/

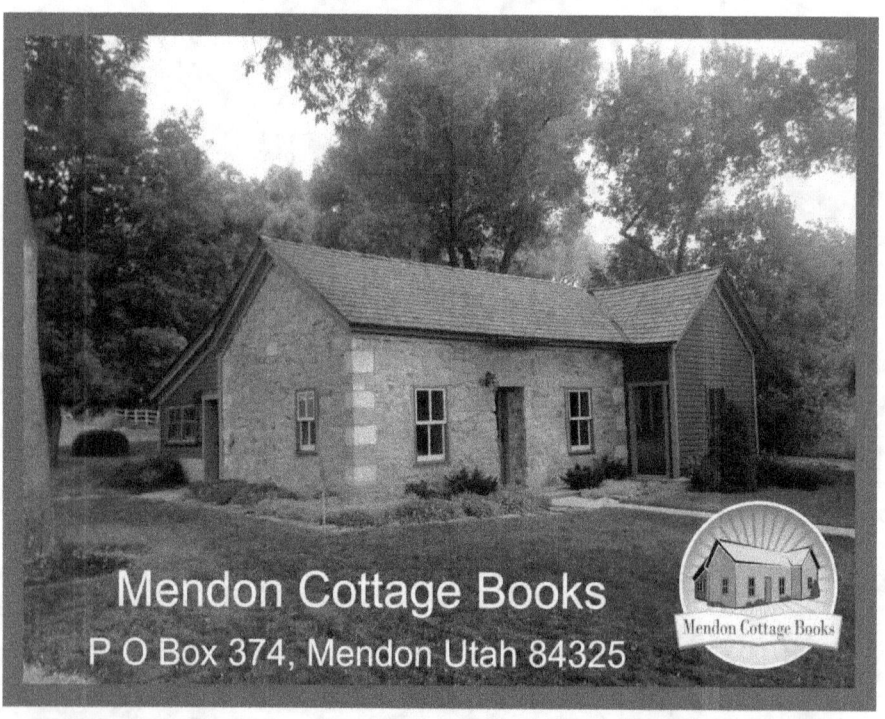

www.ingramcontent.com/pod-product-compliance
Lightning Source LLC
Chambersburg PA
CBHW071144280526
45787CB00003B/1407